Herbal Antibiotics Natural Remedies

Unveiling Nature's Healing Arsenal Discover How to Harness the Potency of 45 Herbal Antibiotics to Combat Any Health Challenge

Jeaneth D. Albert

Published by Jeaneth D. Albert

TABLE OF CONTENTS

Introduction

Medicinal plants are used throughout the world as the source of effective and powerful drugs. Because of the overuse of antibiotics in prescription it leads to the development of antibiotic-resistant strains of bacteria and then they become useless next time so experts are seeing with a hope towards natural and safe antibiotic as alternate. Medicines prepared from the natural herbs are relatively inexpensive and stored for long time at normal temperature. Herbal antibiotics having complex nature which are used to kill bacteria, cleanse blood, enhances immune system and functions of particular organ systems. They work by simply killing bacteria and recover imbalances of body.

Garlic

It is very powerful herb for the treatment of antibiotic-resistant disease. Allicin is the most important active constituent found in garlic which is more powerful than standard

Penicillin. And has excellent antimicrobial functions.

There are different cultures in world recognized garlic as healer and preventive effects because of its antibacterial, antifungal and antiviral properties. Biofilms which act as defence mechanisms of bacteria's and fungus, the allicin inhibits the formation of biofilms because biofilms can makes the treatment of infections very difficult and other active ingredient exist in garlic known as Ajoene that was using in treatment of fungal infections by suppressing bacteria by inhibit the production of enzymes which are responsible for various role of the bacteria such as cell structure formation and energy production and survival of bacteria without energy is impossible. Extract of garlic can also be used for the cure of herpes viruses and influenza and many forms of bacteria like Salmonella and Escherichia coli (E. coli) as a very effective treatment. Garlic is used to reduce blood pressure, enhance immune system, lung and digestive system infections. Garlic was used as antimicrobial agent to prevent gangrene during World Wars. 2.5% of fresh garlic used as a mouth wash and give excellent antimicrobial activity but having Bad breath and unpleasant taste in a recent clinical trial.

Honey

It not having only nutritional value but also having health benefits as a traditional medicine that are used in the curing of tuberculosis, eye diseases, throat infections, bronchial asthma, worm infestation, eczema, constipation, wounds, healing of ulcers. From ancient time honey applied on wounds to heal and prevents infection as antibiotics and nowadays it useful in treating chronic wounds, burns, ulcers, skin sores. The antibacterial effects are due to its hydrogen peroxide content. Wounds infected with methicillin-resistant Staphylococcus aureus treated with honey very effectively by providing a protective coating. The character of honey like as glucose oxidase, hydrogen peroxide, low water acidity and honey prevent the growth of bacteria and yeast. The minimum concentration of honey sufficient for complete inhibitory growth of bacteria. The antibacterial activity of honey is effective against many bacterial pathogens and fungi.

Ginger

It is used as a natural antibiotic. Ginger having the ability to fight against bacteria and helpful in seasickness and nausea and to lower blood sugar levels. Chemical constituents like zingerone, gingerol, terpenoids, zerumbone, gingerdiol, shogaol and flavonoids which gives excellent antimicrobial properties by inhibiting the formation of biofilms. The ginger can normalize the production of acid in stomach so the activity of bacteria H. pylori bacteria grow in stomach in the presence of acid can be reduced acidity by ginger.

Clove

Water extract of clove effective against various kinds of bacteria including E. coli, Staphylococcus aureus, Pseudomonas aeruginosa. Active constituents of clove, eugenol which having excellent antibacterial properties because of having the capacity to destroy the outer layer of bacterial cells by inhibit the production of protein synthesis and it results the inhibition of bacterial growth and in last death of bacteria. Eugenol has antibacterial activity against S. typhi.

Tulsi

Tulsi plant mostly leaf (dried or fresh) are used and mainly three types are commonly found. O. tenuiflorum (or O. sanctum L.) contain two phytochemically and botanically different varieties like Rama tulsi (green leaves) and Shyamatulsi (purplish leaves) and Ocimum gratissimum is another variety of Tulsi called as Vanatulsi (dark green leaves). Tulsi having antibiotics activity against many bacteria like Candida albicans, Staphylococcus aureus, Escherichia coli because of presence of active constituents in it. Ocimum sanctum L. fixed oil having antibacterial activity in which found higher content of linoleic acid in against Pseudomonas aeruginosa, S. aureus and Bacillus pumius, the aqueous extract of Ocimum sanctum L. showed zones of inhibition against Klebsiella. Ursolic acid, Eugenol and carvacrol present in Tulsi possess antimicrobial activity against

Streptococcus mutans. At the 4% concentration level these having maximum antimicrobial activity and enhances immunity and metabolic functions with lowering stress and possessing antioxidant property.

Turmeric

It is a very well-known Indian spice which having antimicrobial properties and flavour. The chemical constituent Curcumin derived from the rhizome of C. longa is an active constituent of turmeric which having very important role in treatment of UTI (Urinary Tract Infections), stomach inflammations as antibacterial as well as antibiofilm activity. Curcumin works as amphipathic and lipophilic so its easily penetrate cell membrane bacteria which results in its leakage and disruption. Due to modulation of gene expression and inhibition of quorum sensing antibiofilm effect shown. It inhibits biofilm and also down regulate many quorum sensing-dependent virulence factors as the production of motility, alginate and swarming.

Rosemary

It acts as effective natural antibiotic without side-effects in salmonella infections and staph infections and much effective in fighting quorum sensing bacteria. The Rosemary oil shown antibacterial activity of against Bacillus cereus, E. coli, Staphylococcus aureus, Salmonella choleraesuis, Aeromonas hydrophila, Bacillus cereus, Staphylococcus aureus and Clostridium perfringens. Active constituents like isorosmanoletc, rosmarinic acid, carnosol, carnosic acid, rosmanol, epirosmanol and rosmaridiphenol work by interaction with the microbial cell membrane that caused change in hereditary material with changing the transport of electrons which results produced the loss of structure and its membrane functionality.

Black cumen

Nigella sativa is herbal plant which is also called black cumen. The seed or it oil also used as a carminative, diuretic, lactagogue and vermifuge from past. It also used in the cure of rheumatic diseases, fever, warts, bites of snake and asthma. Thymoquinone and thymohydroquinone obtained from the

Extraction and isolation of the volatile oil of N. sativa having suppressive activity against gram-negative and gram-positive bacteria. Diethyl ether extract of N. sativa having combining effect with gentamicin and streptomycin exhibit synergetic effect with tobramycin, spectinomycin, erythromycin, nalidixic acid, doxycycline, chloramphenicol, co-trimoxazole, lincomycin, and ampicillin [19]. N. sativa seeds contain oil, protein, saponin, arachidonic acid and carbohydrate. The fixed oil is composed of eicosadenoic acid, linoleic acid, almitoleic acid, palmitic acid, myristic acid, stearic acid, sterols, fiber and oleic acid whereas the essential oil of N. sativa entails nigellone, carvacrol, thymol, α- and β-pinene, p-cymeme, d-limonene, d-citronellol thymoquinone and thymohydroquinone.

Mango

Magnifera indica commonly known as mango belonging to family Anacardiaeceae is the most popular fruit bearing trees in the world. It is a good source of vitamin A. The main active constituents are the polyphenolics, flavonoids, triterpenoids. Mangiferin a xanthone glycoside major bio-active constituent, Seed kernel extract of mango showing inhibitory effect against coliform and E. coli. Trituration of mango kernel or its extract is being used in food products or cosmetics because of its bacteriostatic and antibacterial properties. Acetone leaf extract of mango show antibacterial activity against S. typhi.

The acetone and methanolic extracts reduced the growth of gram-positive bacteria. Bioactive components present in this plant are thermostable. The application of these plant materials requires boiling for long periods but does not affect its efficacy. Temperature stability by plant extracts had earlier been reported in studies.

Onion

Allium cepa is also called as bulb onion or garden onion, and is the widely grown species of the genus Allium. It having powerful flavonoids that have antibiotic effects and contain therapeutic sulfur compounds called cysteine sulphoxides and also having proteins, carbohydrates and phosphorus. If we eat white onion as raw regularly it showed its antioxidant and anti-inflammatory properties. Raw onion is also helpful in reducing swelling from bee stings and onion extract are used in the treatment of topical scars; onion used to treat intestinal infections from ancient time and antibacterial activity was evaluated against V. cholerae. By using disc diffusion method its revealed that Allium sativum was viricidal and had MIC of its aqueous extract is obtained to be 5–15 mg/dl and with acetone extract it was obtained to be 2.5–5 mg/dl. Allium extract considered as a natural preservative or food additive. In addition to its nutritional values it also having the antibacterial activities against lots of both gram-negative and grampositive bacteria including Bacillus subtilis, Salmonella, and E. coli and this inhibiting action also noted on Staphylococcus aureus and results a complete inhibition of all strains tested at a concentration of 6.5mg/ml. Effectiveness in antibacterial activity was depending on the type of onions and extracts concentration. Mostly extracts of onion in concentrations of 50% and it shown excellent antibacterial activity above 50%.

Persian cumin

Carum carvi is also called as Persian cumin belongs to family Apiaceae, mostly contain volatile oil carvone and limonene. The fruits can be used as whole with pungent or anise-like flavor and aroma because of essential oils present in it. C. Carvi is used as antispasmodic, carminative and appetite enhancing agents. C. Carvi essential oils controlled the Gram-positive and Gram-negative bacteria. Caraway essential oil showed the maximum effect on Acinetobacter spp, E. coli, staphylococcus aureus, Proteus spp. and minimum effect on Pseudomonas aeroginosa.

The importance of antibiotics in modern healthcare

The importance of antibiotics in modern healthcare cannot be overstated. These life-saving medications have revolutionized the treatment of bacterial infections and have significantly contributed to improving health outcomes and reducing mortality rates globally. Antibiotics are used not only in the treatment of common infections like urinary tract infections, respiratory tract infections, and skin infections but also in more serious conditions such as sepsis, pneumonia, and meningitis. Antibiotics, by targeting specific bacterial mechanisms, have become a mainstay in treating various infectious diseases. Their mechanism of action ranges from disrupting cell wall synthesis in pathogens like MRSA (Methicillin-resistant Staphylococcus aureus) to inhibiting protein synthesis in gram-negative bacteria.

Concerns about antibiotic resistance

Antibiotic resistance is one of the biggest global issues as bacteria become resistant to the effects of antibiotics and hence are not useful in treating bacterial diseases. This can result in protracted diseases, numerous complications, and fatalities.

Causes of antibiotic resistance include; irrational use of antibiotics, misuse of antibiotics, and antibiotics used in animals. Also, the improper use of antibiotics as well as their abuse leads to the emergence of the resistant bacterial strains.

However, along with the tremendous benefits of antibiotics comes the growing concern of antibiotic resistance. Antibiotic resistance occurs when bacteria develop the ability to evade the effects of antibiotics, rendering these medications ineffective in treating infections. This phenomenon is primarily driven by the overuse and misuse of antibiotics. The misuse of antibiotics can include taking them when they are not needed, not completing a full course of treatment, or taking antibiotics that have been prescribed for someone else.

The rise of herbal antibiotics as an alternative

There are many discussions today on using the herbal antibiotics instead of the traditional antibiotics. As the issue of antibiotic resistance and the side effects of synthetic antibiotics persist, there is a growing emphasis on the use of herbs as cure for infections and enhancing the body's healing mechanisms.

Purpose and scope of the book

At the same time, the goal of the book is to help readers gain extensive knowledge about using herbal antibiotics instead of the traditional antibiotics. It seeks to inform the readers about the importance of using the various types of herbal antibiotics in treating various infections and enhancing the healing process.

The reviewer also pointed out that the book focuses on many types of the herbal antibiotics: familiar ones like garlic, oregano oil, echinacea, and turmeric and other less-known herbs with antimicrobial activity. It further discusses scientific studies of these herbs including their active ingredients and how they affect pathogenic microorganisms.

The book also mentions how the use of herbal antibiotics have been traditional medicine systems including Ayurveda and Traditional Chinese Medicine. This paper gives background knowledge on how these ancient healing practices have relied on use of herbs for infections and their efficiency especially on particular sorts of infections.

In addition, it covers some issues related to the utilization of herbal antibiotics such as the right portion, risks, and compatibility with other drugs. It also stresses the need not to use herbal antibiotics without consulting a doctor especially when one has other health complications or is on other medications.

Furthermore, the author discusses not merely the scientific and medical perspectives but the present role of herbal antibiotics in general healthcare system. It covers the issues of antibiotic resistance and the search for new therapeutic methods. This also explores how herbal antibiotics contribute to overall wellness and the strengthening of the body's defenses.

In summary, the book seeks to educate readers and help them make the right choices in their lives by providing them with crucial information about herbal antibiotics and natural replacements for antibiotics. It is a helpful guide to all people who are concerned with herbal medicine, practitioners who are looking for an alternative approach to treatment, individuals worried about antibiotic resistance and undesirable side effects of synthetic antibiotics.

Chapter 1

Understanding Herbal Antibiotics

Understanding Herbal Antibiotics is related to comprehending how different herbs can be utilized to treat bacterial infections naturally. These fungal antibiotics have been in use for a long time in traditional medicine and they are known to have antimicrobial effects.

Some popular herbal antibiotics are garlic, oregano, echinacea, goldenseal, and turmeric. They can be prepared as teas, tinctures, capsules or ingested directly in food for medicinal purposes.

What are herbal antibiotics?

Herbal antibiotics are plant-derived compounds with antibacterial activity. They can be used instead of conventional antibiotics, which are synthetic medications that treat bacterial infections. Herbal antibiotics have been utilized in traditional health systems around the world for millennia and are still popular today due to their effectiveness and low side effects.

How do they work?

Herbal antibiotics work through various mechanisms to fight against bacteria, viruses, fungi, and other microorganisms. Some herbal antibiotics have direct antimicrobial effects, meaning they can kill or inhibit the growth of harmful microbes. Others work indirectly by boosting the immune system's ability to fight off infections.

Mechanisms of action of herbal antibiotics

There are several mechanisms by which herbal antibiotics exert their antimicrobial effects:

1. Disruption of microbial cell walls: Some herbal antibiotics, such as berberine found in goldenseal and barberry, can disrupt the cell walls of bacteria, making them more susceptible to destruction.

2. Inhibition of bacterial protein synthesis: Herbal antibiotics like tetracycline compounds found in honey and propolis can inhibit the synthesis of proteins in bacterial cells, preventing their growth and replication.

3. Interference with microbial enzymes: Certain herbal antibiotics, such as allicin in garlic and catechins in green tea, can interfere with specific enzymes in microorganisms, disrupting their vital metabolic processes.

4. Modulation of the immune system: Herbal antibiotics like echinacea and astragalus can enhance the functioning of the immune system, making it more effective in fighting infections.

Benefits of herbal antibiotics over conventional antibiotics

There are several benefits to using herbal antibiotics:

1. Reduced risk of antibiotic resistance: Unlike conventional antibiotics, which can contribute to the development of antibiotic-resistant bacteria, herbal antibiotics are less likely to lead to resistance. This is because they contain a complex combination of bioactive compounds that make it difficult for bacteria to develop resistance.

2. Fewer side effects: Herbal antibiotics are generally well-tolerated and have fewer side effects compared to synthetic antibiotics. They are less likely to cause gastrointestinal disturbances, allergic reactions, or disruption of the body's natural microbial balance.

3. Broader spectrum of activity: Many herbal antibiotics have broad-spectrum antimicrobial activity, meaning they can target a wide range of bacteria, viruses, and fungi. This makes them versatile in treating a variety of infections.

4. Support for overall health: In addition to their antimicrobial properties, herbal antibiotics often have other health benefits. For example, garlic has been shown to have antioxidant and anti-inflammatory effects, while turmeric has potent anti-inflammatory and immune-modulating properties.

Safety considerations when using herbal antibiotics

While herbal antibiotics are generally safe, there are some important considerations to keep in mind:

1. Quality and standardization: It is crucial to choose high-quality herbal products from reputable sources to ensure their potency, purity, and safety. Look for standardized extracts that provide a consistent dosage of the active compounds.

2. Drug interactions: Some herbal antibiotics may interact with certain medications, such as blood thinners or immunosuppressants. It is important to consult with a healthcare professional before using herbal antibiotics, especially if you are taking other medications.

3. Allergic reactions: Although rare, some individuals may have allergies or sensitivities to certain herbs. If you experience any adverse reactions, such as itching, rash, or difficulty breathing, discontinue use and seek medical attention.

4. Pregnancy and breastfeeding: Some herbal antibiotics may not be safe for pregnant women or nursing mothers. It is essential to consult with a healthcare professional before using herbal antibiotics during these stages.

5. Dosage and duration of use: Follow the recommended dosage instructions provided by the manufacturer or a healthcare professional. Avoid prolonged or excessive use of herbal antibiotics to prevent potential side effects or imbalances in the body.

In conclusion, herbal antibiotics are natural substances derived from plants that have antimicrobial properties. They work through various mechanisms to kill or inhibit the growth of microorganisms and can be used as an alternative to conventional antibiotics. Herbal antibiotics offer benefits such as reduced risk of antibiotic resistance, fewer side effects, broader spectrum of activity, and added health benefits. However, it is important to consider safety considerations when using herbal antibiotics, including quality and standardization, drug interactions, potential allergies, and appropriate dosage and duration of use. Consulting with a healthcare professional is advised to ensure safe and effective use of herbal antibiotics.

Chapter 2

Choosing the Right Herbal Antibiotics

When it comes to selecting herbal antibiotics, there are several factors to consider. Understanding these factors and the different types of herbal antibiotics available will help you make an informed decision. In this chapter, we will explore these factors and discuss popular herbal antibiotics and their specific uses.

Factors to Consider when Selecting Herbal Antibiotics

1. Type of Infection: Consider the type of infection you are dealing with. Different herbal antibiotics may be more effective against certain types of bacteria, viruses, or fungi. For example, oregano oil is known for its antibacterial properties and is often used for respiratory infections, while tea tree oil is effective against fungal infections like athlete's foot.

2. Potency and Concentration: Look for herbal antibiotics that are standardized and have a consistent potency and concentration. This ensures that you are getting a reliable and effective dose of the active compounds.

3. Quality and Source: Choose herbal antibiotics from reputable sources that prioritize quality and safety. Look for products that are organic, non-GMO, and have undergone third-party testing for purity and potency.

4. Safety and Side Effects: Consider any potential side effects or contraindications of the herbal antibiotic. Some herbs may interact with certain medications or have adverse effects on pre-existing conditions. It is important to consult with a healthcare professional before starting any herbal antibiotic regimen.

5. Personal Preferences: Take into account your personal preferences and ease of use. Some herbal antibiotics are available in different forms such as essential oils, tinctures, teas, capsules, or powders. Choose a form that is convenient and comfortable for you to incorporate into your routine.

Understanding the Different Types of Herbal Antibiotics

1. Essential Oils: Essential oils are concentrated liquids derived from plants and are highly potent. They are often used topically, inhaled, or taken orally under the guidance of a professional. They provide a concentrated dose of the herb's active compounds and are useful for conditions such as skin infections, respiratory infections, and digestive issues.

2. Tinctures: Tinctures are liquid extracts of herbs that are made by steeping the plant material in alcohol or another solvent. They are convenient and easy to use, often taken orally by adding a few drops to water or other beverages. Tinctures are suitable for a wide range of conditions and are particularly effective for urinary tract infections, digestive issues, and immune support.

3. Teas: Herbal teas are made by steeping dried or fresh herbs in hot water. They offer a gentler and milder form of herbal antibiotics. Herbal teas are commonly used for respiratory infections, digestive issues, and as immune boosters. They are also a soothing and comforting way to consume herbs.

4. Capsules and Tablets: Herbal antibiotics in capsule or tablet form are convenient and easy to take. They provide a standardized dosage of the herb's active compounds. Capsules and tablets are suitable for a variety of conditions and are often used for digestive issues, urinary tract infections, and immune support.

Popular Herbal Antibiotics and Their Specific Uses

1. Echinacea: Echinacea is a popular herbal antibiotic known for its immune-enhancing properties. It is commonly used to prevent and treat common colds, influenza, and respiratory infections. Echinacea is available in various forms, including tablets, capsules, tinctures, and teas.

2. Garlic: Garlic is a potent herbal antibiotic with broad-spectrum antimicrobial effects. It is effective against bacteria, viruses, fungi, and parasites. Garlic is often used to support cardiovascular health, boost the immune system, and fight respiratory and digestive infections.

3. Tea Tree Oil: Tea tree oil is a powerful antifungal and antibacterial herbal antibiotic. It is commonly used topically to treat skin infections, such as acne, athlete's foot, and nail fungus. Tea tree oil can be applied directly to the affected area or diluted in a carrier oil.

4. Goldenseal: Goldenseal is a well-known herbal antibiotic that contains the active compound berberine. It has potent antimicrobial effects and is commonly used to treat respiratory and digestive infections, urinary tract infections, and skin conditions.

5. Olive Leaf Extract: Olive leaf extract is a natural antibiotic with broad-spectrum antimicrobial properties. It is effective against bacteria, viruses, fungi, and parasites. Olive leaf extract is commonly used to strengthen the immune system, fight infections, and support cardiovascular health.

In conclusion, choosing the right herbal antibiotics involves considering factors such as the type of infection, potency and concentration, quality and source, safety and side effects, and personal preferences. Understanding the different types of herbal antibiotics, including essential oils, tinctures, teas, capsules, and tablets, is important for selecting the most suitable form. Popular herbal antibiotics like echinacea, garlic, tea tree oil, goldenseal, and olive leaf extract have specific uses and are effective against various types of infections. Consulting with a healthcare professional will ensure that you choose the most appropriate herbal antibiotics for your specific needs.

Chapter 3

Garlic

Garlic has been used for centuries not only as a flavoring agent in various cuisines but also for its medicinal properties. This versatile herb is known for its distinctive aroma and taste, but it also offers several health benefits. In this chapter, we will explore the health benefits of garlic, the component responsible for its antibacterial properties, and how to use garlic as a natural antibiotic. Additionally, we will provide some recipes and remedies that incorporate garlic.

Health Benefits of Garlic

Garlic is packed with several vital nutrients, including vitamins, minerals, and antioxidants, which contribute to its numerous health benefits. Some of the key advantages of including garlic in your diet are:

1. Boosts Immunity: Garlic helps to strengthen the immune system, making it effective in fighting off common illnesses like the flu and colds.

2. Lowers Blood Pressure: Allicin, a compound found in garlic, helps relax blood vessels, thus reducing blood pressure levels. This can be beneficial in preventing cardiovascular diseases.

3. Reduces Cholesterol Levels: Regular consumption of garlic has been linked to lowering LDL cholesterol (known as the "bad" cholesterol) levels, reducing the risk of heart disease.

4. Antioxidant Properties: Garlic contains antioxidants that help protect the body against damage caused by free radicals, reducing the risk of chronic diseases such as cancer.

Allicin and Its Antibacterial Properties

Allicin, the main active compound found in garlic, is responsible for many of its health benefits, particularly its antibacterial properties. When garlic is crushed or chopped, it releases allicin, which has demonstrated antimicrobial activity against various bacteria, including antibiotic-resistant strains.

A study published in the Journal of Antimicrobial Chemotherapy found that allicin effectively killed bacteria such as Staphylococcus aureus and Escherichia coli. Its antibacterial properties make garlic a natural alternative to synthetic antibiotics.

Using Garlic as an Antibiotic

Garlic can be used as a natural antibiotic in various ways. Here are a few methods to incorporate garlic into your routine:

1. Raw Garlic: Consuming raw garlic cloves daily can help fight bacterial infections. Start by crushing or mincing a clove of garlic and letting it sit for a few minutes to activate the beneficial compounds. Then, either eat it directly or mix it with honey or olive oil for easier consumption.

2. Garlic Infused Oil: Infusing garlic into oil creates a potent antibacterial mixture. Simply crush a few garlic cloves and add them to a bottle of olive oil. Allow it to sit for a week, shaking occasionally. You can then use this oil in cooking or incorporate it into dressings or sauces.

3. Garlic Capsules: Garlic supplements in the form of capsules or pills are available in most health stores. These supplements are standardized for allicin content and provide a convenient way to obtain the benefits of garlic regularly.

Recipes and Remedies Using Garlic

Garlic can be used in numerous culinary creations and home remedies. Here are a few recipes and remedies showcasing the versatility of garlic:

1. Roasted Garlic Soup: Roast a head of garlic in the oven until soft and golden. Squeeze out the roasted cloves and blend them with vegetable broth, onions, and other desired spices. Simmer until heated through and enjoy a nourishing and flavorsome soup.

How to cook Roasted Garlic Soup

This recipe uses over 40 cloves of garlic. And it's the perfect amount to produce a subtle garlic flavor that's richly creamy. Some of the cloves get roasted ahead of time in the oven; you can do this a day ahead of time. And the rest are simmered until soft in the broth. Since the garlic gets cooked to softness, this takes the edge off the sharp garlic flavor of raw or flash-sautee'd garlic. If you like some garlic with bite, feel free to garnish the soup with some raw cloves that have been minced.

Ingredients

- 26 garlic cloves, peeled
- 2 Tablespoons olive oil
- 2 Tablespoons butter
- 2 medium onions, sliced (about 2 generous cups)
- 2 teaspoons chopped fresh thyme, or ½ teaspoon dried
- 18 garlic cloves, smashed and peeled

- 4 cups chicken broth, low-sodium or vegetable broth
- ½ cup whipping cream, half and half, oat or almond milk work well
- ½ teaspoon sea salt
- ½ teaspoon freshly ground black pepper
- ½ cup finely grated Parmesan cheese
- 1 large russet potato, not peeled, cut into large chunks (optional)
- 4 lemon wedges

Optional variations and other garnishes-see instructions for how to incorporate:

- Toasted croutons, drizzled in oil, salt and pepper then baked at 350F degrees until golden
- 8 cloves fresh garlic, minced and sauteed just until fragrant in olive oil, dashed with pepper
- Parmesan Crisps, *recipe below*

Instructions

Make the roasted garlic, this can be done a day ahead:

1. Preheat the oven to 350F degrees. Cut the bottom portion off where the garlic attaches to the base. To make peeling the garlic easy, you can smash them a bit then the peel will come right off. Place garlic in small glass baking dish. Drizzle with 2 Tablespoons olive oil and add a dash each of salt and pepper. Toss to coat. Cover baking dish tightly with a lid or foil and bake until garlic is golden brown and tender, about 45 minutes. Transfer cloves to small bowl. If making the day before, place cooled garlic in a plastic bag or covered dish and refrigerate until needed. By the way, this roasted garlic is fabulous anytime for a garlic paste or just for snacking on the roasted garlic cloves. The oil, salt and pepper, and roasting method create a fabulous treat.

Make the soup

1. Melt 2 Tablespoons butter in a heavy, large saucepan over medium-high heat.

2. Add 2 onions and 2 teaspoons thyme and cook until onions are translucent, about 5 minutes.

3. Add roasted garlic and 18 raw garlic cloves and cook a couple of minutes to release some of the raw garlic oils.

4. If you're adding the russet potato chunks, add now as well.

5. Add 4 cups chicken or vegetable broth; cover and simmer until garlic is very tender, about 20 minutes. If you're making the Parmesan Cheese Crisps, make them now while the soup is simmering.

6. If you added the russet potato chunks, remove them after the 20 minute simmer and place in a small bowl or on a plate while you puree the rest of the ingredients. Working in batches, puree soup in a blender until smooth or puree with an immersion blender. Return potato chunks to the creamed soup.

7. Return soup to the saucepan, add ½ cup cream, or whatever milk you are using, and bring to a very low simmer just to reheat, being careful not to

curdle the milk. Add ½ teaspoon salt and ½ teaspoon freshly ground pepper. Taste and add more to your liking.

8. Divide the grated ½ cup of Parmesan cheese among 4 bowls and ladle soup over. Each bowl will get about 2 tablespoons of cheese.

9. Squeeze juice of 1 lemon wedge into each bowl and serve.

10. Serve in individual bowls garnished with more grated Parmesan, Parmesan Crips or toasted croutons, or the additional minced sauteed garlic.

How to make the Parmesan Crisp Garnish:

1. Heat your oven to 400F degrees, Pour a heaping Tablespoon of grated Parmesan onto a silicone or parchment lined baking sheet and pat down just a bit. For color or extra flavor, you could sprinkle the cheese mound with herbs, black pepper or red pepper flakes. Repeat with as much Parmesan crisps as desired, spacing the spoonfuls about a ½ inch

apart. Bake until golden and crisp. Since ovens vary, this time can be anywhere from 3 to 10 minutes (mine finished closer to the 10 minute mark). The cheese will bubble quite a bit, but just keep cooking until the crisps darken. Cool, then using a spatula, carefully scrape the crips off the baking sheet and serve with the soup.

Notes

- The roasted garlic can be made a day ahead of making the soup and this method for roasting garlic creates delicious little garlic nuggets to enjoy for any reason or to make a garlic paste for hearty bread.
- The recipe is doubled easily and can be refrigerated for 2 or 3 days before serving.

2. Garlic Honey Cough Syrup: Crush a few cloves of garlic and mix them with raw honey. Allow the mixture to sit for a few hours to infuse. Take a spoonful of this syrup as needed to soothe a cough or sore throat.

Garlic honey cough syrup is a natural remedy that combines the antibacterial and antiviral properties of garlic with the soothing and healing properties of honey. Here is a simple recipe for making garlic honey cough syrup:

Ingredients:

- 3-4 cloves of garlic
- 1/2 cup raw honey

Instructions:

1. Peel and crush the garlic cloves.
2. Place the crushed garlic in a clean glass jar.
3. Pour honey over the garlic, making sure it is completely covered.
4. Seal the jar and let it sit for at least 24 hours to allow the garlic to infuse into the honey.
5. Take 1 teaspoon of the syrup as needed to help relieve cough and sore throat.

Never give honey to a child under 1 year of age.

1. Fill a small clean jar with peeled garlic cloves
2. Pour raw honey over top
3. Push the cloves down to ensure the garlic is covered with honey
4. Put a lid on and leave overnight for at least 12 hours.
5. Store in the cupboard. After two weeks, remove the garlic cloves.
6. Take a spoonful of the honey garlic as needed for coughs and sore throats.

If you don't have time to wait 12 hours, just crush a clove of garlic, mix with honey and eat that - it'll have a stronger flavor but equally effective (as long as the garlic is crushed or chewed!)

3. Garlic and Herb Roasted Chicken: Crush garlic cloves, mix them with herbs such as rosemary and thyme, and rub the mixture all over a chicken before roasting. This simple yet delicious recipe provides a flavorful and healthy meal.

Ingredients to make this roasted chicken recipe

Herbs: We are using fresh rosemary sprigs, parsley and thyme here and making our chicken blend with extra-virgin olive oil and fresh grated garlic, and of course seasoning with kosher salt and black pepper!

Chicken: I love a whole spatchcocked chicken, and that's what we are using here. Feel free to use a whole chicken as well without the backbone removed, but keep in mind roasted time may be longer.

Garlic and lemon: Whole garlic and lemon are being roasted with the chicken, where they are then squeezed over the finished chicken.

Option to add on any of your favorite vegetables here in the roasting pan as well such as potatoes, carrots, onion or celery! You can also add on a herb butter, too to roast with this chicken.

Instructions to make this recipe

Dry brine your chicken

- Pat your chicken dry with paper towels. Season with kosher salt and freshly ground black pepper on all sides and inside the chicken cavity. Place on a large sheet tray lined with parchment paper and dry brine for 2 hours or overnight in the fridge, without covering. Skip this step if you are not dry-brining!
- You don't have to dry brine; however, this allows the flavors to infuse, the chicken to become more tender, and allows drying out the chicken skin to ensure the extra crispness of the skin!

Season and roast your chicken

1. When your chicken is ready to roast, preheat your oven to 425 degrees, convection if you have it. In a small bowl, mix together your extra-virgin olive oil, parsley, thyme, rosemary and grated garlic. Season with kosher salt and black pepper. Mix well until incorporated.
2. In a large baking dish or large cast iron that will fit your chicken fully, place your chicken in, and add in your

head of garlic (halved) and your lemon (halved) around the chicken. Pour over your herb mixture and make sure it's coating all over the chicken. Pat well and spread around until evenly distributed all across the bird.

3. Place in the preheated oven and roast for 40 to 50 minutes, until crispy on the outside and cooked fully on the inside (it should be 165 degrees at the thickest part of the breast when using a meat thermometer), until the juices run clear when you cut between leg and thigh.

4. Halfway through the cooking time, you can also baste some of the liquid on top of the bird. I also rotated my pan halfway through cooking to get even crispiness on all sides.

Carve and serve

1. When fully cooked, remove, and let rest for about 15 minutes to prepare for carving your chicken. Carve, plate and pour over any remaining pan juices.

Ingredients

- 4 to 5 pound whole spatchcocked chicken
- kosher salt and freshly ground black pepper
- 1/4 cup extra-virgin olive oil
- 1 tablespoon dried parsley
- 1 tablespoon dried thyme
- 1 tablespoon fresh rosemary, finely chopped
- 4 garlic cloves, minced or grated
- 1 head of garlic, halved
- 1 whole large lemon, halved

Instructions

1. Pat your chicken dry with paper towels. Season with kosher salt and freshly ground black pepper on all sides and inside the chicken cavity. Place on a large sheet tray lined with parchment paper and dry brine for 2 hours or overnight in the fridge, without covering. Skip this step if you are not dry-brining!
   You don't have to dry brine; however, this allows the flavors to infuse, the

chicken to become more tender, and allows drying out the chicken skin to ensure the extra crispness of the skin!

2. When your chicken is ready to roast, preheat your oven to 425 degrees, convection if you have it. In a small bowl, mix together your extra-virgin olive oil, parsley, thyme, rosemary and grated garlic. Season with kosher salt and black pepper. Mix well until incorporated.

3. In a large baking dish or large cast iron that will fit your chicken fully, place your chicken in, and add in your head of garlic (halved) and your lemon (halved) around the chicken. Pour over your herb mixture and make sure it's coating all over the chicken. Pat well and spread around until evenly distributed all across the bird.

4. Place in the preheated oven and roast for 40 to 50 minutes, until crispy on the outside and cooked fully on the inside (it should be 165 degrees at the thickest part of the breast when using

a meat thermometer), until the juices run clear when you cut between leg and thigh.

Halfway through the cooking time, you can also baste some of the liquid on top of the bird. I also rotated my pan halfway through cooking to get even crispiness on all sides.

5. When fully cooked, remove, and let rest for about 15 minutes. Carve, plate, and pour over any remaining pan juices, in addition to including a squeeze of the lemon and roasted garlic that has been cooked and charred with the chicken.

In conclusion, garlic offers a range of health benefits due to its abundance of nutrients and the presence of allicin, which possesses powerful antibacterial properties. Whether consumed raw, infused in oil, or taken in supplement form, garlic can be used as a natural antibiotic to fight off infections. Additionally, garlic can be incorporated into various recipes and home remedies, making it a versatile ingredient in both the kitchen and the medicine cabinet.

Chapter 4

Echinacea

Echinacea is a popular herbal remedy that has been used for centuries to boost the immune system and treat various ailments. This chapter will provide an overview of echinacea, its immune-boosting and antibiotic properties, different forms and preparations of echinacea, and dosage recommendations.

Overview of Echinacea

Echinacea, also known as coneflower, is a flowering plant native to North America. It is a part of the daisy family and has been widely used in traditional medicine by Native American tribes. Echinacea is renowned for its immune-stimulating properties and has been extensively studied for its potential benefits in supporting the body's natural defenses.

Echinacea as an Immune Booster and Antibiotic

One of the primary uses of echinacea is as an immune booster. It stimulates the activity of various immune cells, such as T-cells and natural killer cells, which play a crucial role in fighting off infections. Echinacea also enhances the production of cytokines, which are signaling molecules that regulate immune responses.

In addition to its immune-boosting effects, echinacea also exhibits antibiotic properties. It can help inhibit the growth of certain bacteria, such as Streptococcus and Staphylococcus, making it a valuable natural alternative to synthetic antibiotics.

Different Forms and Preparations of Echinacea

Echinacea is available in various forms, including:

1. Echinacea Tea: Echinacea tea is made by steeping the aerial parts of the plant, such as the flowers and leaves, in hot water. It is a convenient and common way to consume echinacea. To prepare echinacea tea, simply add one teaspoon of dried echinacea herb per cup of hot water and steep for 10-15 minutes. You can drink this tea three to four times a day.

How to Make Echinacea Tea

Echinacea tea can be made from the echinacea root or flowers of your garden plant. You can use fresh flowers, leaves, stems, and roots, or dry a batch to always have some on hand. Here well give you a basic recipe to brew echinacea herb tea at home.

Basic Echinacea tea Recipe

Ingredients:

- 1 tablespoon dried echinacea (or 2 tablespoons of fresh echinacea)
- 10 ounces of water
- Sweetener (OPTIONAL)

Instructions:

1. Bring water to a boil using a stove-top pan or a tea kettle.

2. Once boiling, turn the heat down to medium and add in the echinacea.
3. Place a lid on the pot and simmer for 5 to 10 minutes. If using a tea kettle, simply pour the boiling water into a teacup and add the echinacea to a tea ball or tea infuser. Steep for 5 to 10 minutes.
4. Strain the loose flowers, roots, or leaves from the pot and pour into a teacup. It using a tea ball, simply remove and discard the echinacea.
5. Add flavorings or sweeteners such as honey and lemon if desired. Enjoy!

2. Echinacea Tincture: Echinacea tincture is made by extracting the active compounds from the plant using alcohol or glycerin. This concentrated form allows for easy dosage adjustments. Tinctures can be consumed by adding a few drops to water or juice.

How to Make Herb Tincture

Echinacea tincture is one of my go-to herbal remedies for colds and flu. This powerful remedy makes a fantastic addition to home apothecaries and first aid kits. Learning how to make it will save you money and empower the health of you and your loved ones.

Note: if you're excited about making a shelf stable Echinacea extract but don't want to use alcohol, you can use vegetable glycerine instead. In the ingredients list below I've included this substitution option. With the glycerine, you'll follow the same directions but just use glycerine instead of vodka.

What you'll need...

- 150 grams dried cut/sifted Echinacea angustifolia root (approximately 1 ½ cups)
- 750 ml 100 proof vodka (or for a non-alcohol version, substitute this with 500 ml glycerine and 250 ml water)\

Instructions

1. Place the Echinacea root in a quart jar
2. Pour the vodka over the Echinacea root.

3. Cover the jar with a lid and shake well. Continue to shake the jar everyday for 1 week and then every few days while its macerating (extracting) over the next 6 weeks.

4. You'll notice that the Echinacea root will expand as it soaks up the alcohol. If the roots expand so much that the alcohol no longer covers them, add a bit more vodka. However, you want to add as little as possible to avoid diluting the mixture too much.

5. After 6 weeks, give the jar one last really good shake. Then strain the roots through cheesecloth, squeezing it well. (Alternatively use a potato ricer to strain and squeeze the roots.)

6. Using a small funnel, pour the tincture into clean dropper bottles. Store in a cool, dark place.

Yield: 2 ¾ cups tincture

3. Echinacea Capsules or Tablets: Echinacea is also available in capsule or tablet form. This provides a more convenient and standardized way of consuming echinacea. Follow the dosage instructions provided on the packaging or consult a healthcare professional for guidance.

Dosage Recommendations:

The appropriate dosage of echinacea may vary depending on the individual and the specific product being used. It is advisable to follow the instructions provided by the manufacturer or consult a healthcare professional for personalized guidance. However, general dosage recommendations for echinacea are as follows:

1. **Echinacea Tea:** Drink three to four cups of echinacea tea per day, especially at the onset of symptoms or during periods of immune challenges.

2. **Echinacea Tincture:** Take 2-3 mL (approximately 40-60 drops) of echinacea tincture diluted in water or juice three times daily.

3. **Echinacea Capsules or Tablets:** Follow the dosage guidelines provided on the product packaging. Typically, the

recommended dosage is 300-500 mg, taken two to three times daily.

It is important to note that echinacea should not be taken continuously for long periods. It is typically recommended to take echinacea for a maximum of 10 consecutive days, followed by a break of a few weeks before resuming if necessary.

In conclusion, echinacea is a well-known herbal remedy with immune-boosting and antibiotic properties. It can be consumed in various forms, such as tea, tincture, capsules, or tablets. The appropriate dosage of echinacea may vary, so it is essential to follow the instructions provided or consult a healthcare professional for personalized advice. Echinacea can be a valuable addition to your natural medicine cabinet to support overall immune health and combat common infections.

Chapter 5

Goldenrod

Goldenrod is a flowering plant that belongs to the Asteraceae family. It is native to North America, Europe, and Asia and is known for its vibrant golden-yellow flowers. Goldenrod has a long history of traditional use for various health conditions, particularly as an antibiotic. This chapter will explore the properties and uses of goldenrod as an antibiotic, its preparation as goldenrod tea and other remedies, as well as safety precautions and contraindications.

Properties and Uses of Goldenrod as an Antibiotic:

Goldenrod contains several active compounds that contribute to its antibiotic properties. These include saponins, flavonoids, tannins, and volatile oils. These compounds have been found to have antimicrobial activity against a wide range of bacteria, including strains that are resistant to conventional antibiotics.

Goldenrod has been traditionally used to treat urinary tract infections (UTIs), respiratory infections, and skin infections. Its antibiotic properties help fight off harmful bacteria and support the body's natural defense mechanisms. Goldenrod extracts may also have anti-inflammatory effects, which can aid in the healing process.

Goldenrod Tea and Other Remedies:

Goldenrod tea is one of the most popular ways to consume goldenrod for its antibiotic benefits. To prepare goldenrod tea, steep 1-2 teaspoons of dried goldenrod flowers and leaves in a cup of boiling water for about 10 minutes. Strain and drink the tea two to three times a day.

Apart from goldenrod tea, a tincture can also be made using alcohol or glycerin to extract the beneficial compounds from the plant. A few drops of the tincture can be added to water or juice and consumed as needed.

Goldenrod extracts are also available in the form of capsules or tablets, providing a more convenient and standardized way of consumption. Follow the dosage instructions provided on the product packaging or consult a healthcare professional for personalized guidance.

How to Make Goldenrod Tea

Step 1: Cut off the tops of a few goldenrod flowers. The amount you need is related to both the amount you want to make, as well as how intense you would like the flavor to be. This is all individual preference, practice makes perfect!

Step 2: Chop it all up so it fits in the pot nicely!

Step 3: Toss the flowers (leaves and stems are OK too) into a pot and pour in some water. The water amount is again related to personal preference. I like to use about 1000 liters of water (because it fills a mason jar perfectly) and 3 or 4 robust goldenrod flower crowns. This makes for a potent tea!

Step 4: Bring the water to a boil and then turn off the heat and take the pot off the burner. Let the flowers steep for around 30 minutes.

Step 5: Pour through a fine mesh strainer and enjoy your goldenrod tea!

Safety Precautions and Contraindications:

While goldenrod is generally safe for most individuals when consumed in the recommended amounts, it is essential to exercise caution and be aware of potential contraindications.

Some individuals may be allergic to goldenrod and may experience allergic reactions, such as skin rashes or respiratory symptoms, when exposed to the plant. If you have a known allergy to other plants in the Asteraceae family (such as ragweed, daisies, or marigolds), it is advisable to avoid goldenrod or consult with a healthcare professional before use.

Goldenrod may also have diuretic properties, which can increase urinary output. If you have kidney or bladder issues, it is recommended to consult a healthcare professional before using goldenrod as it may interfere with certain medications or exacerbate existing conditions.

Pregnant and breastfeeding women should also exercise caution and seek medical advice before using goldenrod, as there is limited research on its safety in these populations.

In conclusion, goldenrod is a flowering plant with antibiotic properties that have been traditionally used for various health conditions. Goldenrod tea, tinctures, capsules, and tablets are popular forms of consuming goldenrod for its antibiotic benefits. However, it is essential to consider safety precautions and be aware of any contraindications, such as allergies or existing health conditions, before using goldenrod. If you are unsure about its suitability for your specific situation, it is recommended to consult a healthcare professional for personalized advice.

Chapter 6

Thyme

Thyme is a perennial herb that belongs to the mint family, Lamiaceae. It is native to the Mediterranean region but is now cultivated worldwide. Thyme has a long history of use in culinary and medicinal applications, thanks to its distinct flavor and numerous health benefits. This chapter will explore the antibacterial and antifungal properties of thyme, its uses in cooking and medicine, recipes and remedies utilizing thyme, and potential side effects of thyme consumption.

Antibacterial and Antifungal Properties of Thyme

Thyme contains essential oils such as thymol, carvacrol, and terpinene-4-ol, which contribute to its impressive antibacterial and antifungal properties. These compounds have been shown to inhibit the growth of various bacteria and fungi, including those that are resistant to conventional antibiotics.

The antimicrobial properties of thyme make it an effective natural alternative for treating infections. Thyme oil or extracts derived from thyme can be used topically to treat skin infections, such as acne or athlete's foot. Additionally, thyme can be used internally to combat oral infections, digestive tract infections, and respiratory infections.

Culinary and Medicinal Applications of Thyme

Thyme is a versatile herb that adds a fragrant and earthy flavor to a wide range of dishes. It is commonly used in Mediterranean, Middle Eastern, and European cuisines. Thyme pairs well with meats, stews, soups, roasted vegetables, and marinades. It can be used fresh or dried, but the essential oils are more potent in fresh thyme.

Beyond its culinary uses, thyme also has medicinal applications. It has been traditionally used to relieve respiratory conditions such as coughs, bronchitis, and asthma. Thyme tea can be made by steeping fresh or dried thyme leaves in hot water for about 10 minutes. This tea can help soothe sore throats and reduce coughing. Thyme oil can also be used in steam inhalation to alleviate congestion.

Recipes and Remedies using Thyme

1. **Thyme Infused Honey:** Combine fresh thyme sprigs with honey in a jar and let it infuse for a few days. This infused honey can be used as a natural cough syrup or added to hot tea for soothing relief.

2. **Thyme Roasted Vegetables:** Toss a mixture of chopped vegetables, such as potatoes, carrots, onions, and zucchini, with olive oil, salt, pepper, and fresh thyme leaves. Roast in the oven until tender and golden.

3. **Thyme Facial Steam:** Boil water in a pot, remove from heat, and add a handful of fresh thyme leaves. Cover your head with a towel and lean over the pot, allowing the steam to gently

cleanse your face. This can help open up pores and clear congested skin.

Potential Side Effects of Thyme Consumption

Thyme is generally safe for consumption in the recommended amounts, but some people may experience certain side effects or allergic reactions. These can include gastrointestinal upset or skin irritation. It is essential to use thyme in moderation and discontinue use if any adverse reactions occur.

Thyme may also interact with certain medications, such as blood thinners, anticoagulants, or antihypertensive drugs. If you are taking any medications or have underlying health conditions, it is advisable to consult with a healthcare professional before incorporating thyme into your diet or using it medicinally.

Additionally, individuals with allergies to other plants in the Lamiaceae family, including basil, mint, or oregano, may also be allergic to thyme. It is important to exercise caution and discontinue use if any allergic symptoms arise.

In conclusion, thyme is a versatile herb with potent antibacterial and antifungal properties. It can be used in culinary applications to enhance the flavor of various dishes, as well as in medicinal applications to alleviate respiratory conditions and treat infections. Thyme-infused remedies, such as honey or facial steams, can provide additional health benefits. However, it is important to be aware of potential side effects and consult a healthcare professional when necessary.

Chapter 7

Oregano

Oregano, also known as Origanum vulgare, is a popular herb that is widely used in cooking for its distinct flavor and aroma. However, beyond its culinary applications, oregano also possesses numerous health benefits. In this chapter, we will delve into the different aspects of oregano, including its antimicrobial effects, medicinal uses, recipes, and remedies, as well as precautions when using oregano oil.

The antimicrobial effects of oregano:

Oregano is renowned for its potent antimicrobial properties. It contains compounds such as carvacrol and thymol, which have been found to exhibit strong antimicrobial activity against various pathogens, including bacteria, viruses, and fungi. Research has shown that these compounds can inhibit the growth of pathogenic microorganisms and help in preventing infections. Oregano's antimicrobial effects make it a valuable natural alternative to conventional antibiotics and antifungals.

Oregano oil and other forms of oregano for medicinal use:

Oregano oil, derived from the leaves and flowers of the oregano plant, is one of the most popular forms of oregano used for medicinal purposes. It is highly concentrated and provides a more potent dose of the herb's beneficial compounds. Oregano oil is commonly used to alleviate respiratory conditions, such as coughs, colds, and bronchitis, due to its antimicrobial and expectorant properties.

Apart from oregano oil, other forms of oregano, including dried oregano leaves and oregano tea, can also be used for medicinal purposes. Dried oregano leaves are often incorporated into herbal remedies to boost the immune system, relieve digestive issues, and reduce inflammation. Oregano tea is a soothing beverage that can effectively alleviate sore throats, indigestion, and menstrual cramps.

Recipes and remedies incorporating oregano

Oregano is a versatile herb that can be incorporated into numerous recipes and remedies. In culinary applications, it is commonly used in Italian and Mediterranean cuisines to enhance the flavors of soups, stews, sauces, and marinades. Oregano can also be sprinkled on top of pizzas, added to salads, or used as a garnish for savory dishes.

In terms of remedies, oregano can be used to prepare herbal infusions, or simply added to boiling water to create a steam inhalation for respiratory relief. Oregano essential oil can be applied topically, in diluted form, to treat skin infections, acne, and muscle aches. Additionally, oregano can be combined with other herbs and spices to create herbal blends for teas, tinctures, and capsules.

Precautions when using oregano oil

While oregano and oregano oil provide a range of health benefits, it's important to use them with caution. Oregano oil is highly concentrated and should be diluted before use to avoid skin irritation or sensitivities. It is advisable to perform a patch test before applying oregano oil topically. Furthermore, pregnant women, breastfeeding mothers, and individuals with allergies or sensitive stomachs should consult with a healthcare professional before using oregano oil or consuming large amounts of oregano as a herbal supplement.

In conclusion, oregano is not only a flavorful herb but also a valuable medicinal plant. Its antimicrobial effects, particularly through oregano oil, make it an effective natural remedy for various health conditions. From culinary applications to herbal remedies, oregano offers versatile benefits. However, precautions should be taken when using oregano oil to ensure safe and effective usage.

Chapter 8

Ginger

Ginger, scientifically known as Zingiber officinale, is a root spice that has been used for centuries for its medicinal properties and unique flavor. In this chapter, we will explore the various health benefits of ginger, its role as an antibacterial agent, different ways to use ginger as an antibiotic, and guidelines for ginger consumption.

Health benefits of ginger

Ginger is packed with bioactive compounds that contribute to its numerous health benefits. It is known for its anti-inflammatory, antioxidant, and digestive properties. Some of the key health benefits associated with ginger consumption include:

- **Relieving nausea and morning sickness:** Ginger has long been used as a natural remedy for combating nausea and vomiting.

It is especially helpful for pregnant women experiencing morning sickness.

- **Reducing muscle pain and soreness:** The anti-inflammatory properties of ginger can help alleviate muscle pain and soreness caused by exercise or certain medical conditions.

- **Easing digestion:** Ginger aids in digestion by increasing the production of digestive enzymes, reducing inflammation in the gut, and improving gut motility.

- **Managing chronic diseases:** Ginger has been shown to have potential benefits in managing conditions such as osteoarthritis, diabetes, and cardiovascular disease due to its anti-inflammatory and antioxidant effects.

Ginger as an antibacterial agent

In addition to its well-known health benefits, ginger also possesses antibacterial properties. Research suggests that ginger extract can inhibit the growth of various bacteria, including those responsible for respiratory infections, food poisoning, and periodontal diseases. The antibacterial activity of ginger is attributed to its bioactive compounds, such as gingerols and shogaols.

Ways to use ginger as an antibiotic

Ginger can be used in various forms to harness its antibacterial effects. Here are a few ways to incorporate ginger into your routine as a natural antibiotic:

- **Fresh ginger:** Adding freshly grated or sliced ginger to your meals, such as stir-fries, soups, or marinades, can provide a flavorful antibacterial boost.

- **Ginger tea:** Brewing ginger slices in hot water to create a warm and soothing ginger tea is a popular way to enjoy the antibacterial properties of ginger.

- **Ginger juice:** Extracting the juice from fresh ginger can be used in smoothies, salad dressings, or consumed on its own for a potent antibacterial dose.

- **Ginger capsules:** Ginger supplements in the form of capsules or tablets can provide a standardized dosage of ginger extract for consistent antibacterial benefits.

Dosage guidelines for ginger consumption

When consuming ginger for its antibacterial effects, it's essential to consider the appropriate dosage to ensure safety and efficacy. The recommended dosage of ginger can vary depending on the purpose and individual needs. Here are some general guidelines:

- **Fresh ginger:** 1-2 grams (around half an inch of fresh ginger) per day is a commonly recommended dosage for general health benefits.

- **Ginger tea:** 2-4 cups of ginger tea per day is usually considered safe and effective.

- **Ginger supplements:** Follow the recommended dosage on the product label or consult with a healthcare professional for personalized guidance.

It's important to note that excessive consumption of ginger may cause digestive discomfort, including heartburn or acid reflux. Pregnant women, individuals with bleeding disorders, or those taking blood-thinning medications should consult with a healthcare professional before significantly increasing their ginger intake.

In conclusion, ginger not only adds a delightful flavor to dishes but also offers a multitude of health benefits. Its antibacterial properties make it a valuable natural antibiotic. Incorporating ginger in various forms, such as fresh ginger, ginger tea, ginger juice, or ginger supplements, can help harness its antibacterial effects. However, it's crucial to follow dosage guidelines and consult with a healthcare professional if needed to ensure safe and appropriate use of ginger.

Chapter 9

Turmeric

Turmeric, also known as Curcuma longa, is a vibrant yellow-orange spice commonly used in Indian and Asian cuisines. It has gained much popularity in recent years due to its numerous health benefits, particularly its powerful antibiotic properties. In this chapter, we will explore the various aspects of turmeric, including how to incorporate it into your daily routine, the different turmeric-based remedies and recipes available, as well as potential interactions and contraindications to be aware of.

One of the most notable health benefits of turmeric is its antibiotic properties. This ancient spice has been used for centuries as an effective natural remedy for various ailments and infections. It contains a compound called curcumin, which has been found to exhibit antimicrobial activity against a wide range of bacteria, viruses, fungi, and parasites. The antibacterial properties of turmeric make it a useful addition to your natural medicine cabinet.

The Powerful Antibiotic Properties of Turmeric

Turmeric (Curcuma longa) has been celebrated for centuries for its medicinal properties. The active compound in turmeric, curcumin, is known for its potent antibacterial, antiviral, antifungal, and anti-inflammatory effects. Research has shown that curcumin can inhibit the growth of various bacteria, including Staphylococcus aureus, Escherichia coli, and Helicobacter pylori. This makes turmeric an effective natural remedy for preventing and treating infections.

Mechanisms of Action

1. **Inhibition of Bacterial Growth:** Curcumin disrupts bacterial cell membranes and interferes with their ability to replicate.
2. **Anti-inflammatory Effects:** By reducing inflammation, curcumin

helps the immune system function more effectively.

3. **Antioxidant Properties:** Curcumin scavenges free radicals, protecting cells from damage and boosting overall immunity.

How to Incorporate Turmeric into Your Daily Routine

Incorporating turmeric into your daily routine can be simple and enjoyable. Here are several ways to add this powerful spice to your diet and lifestyle:

Dietary Incorporation

1. **Golden Milk:** Mix 1 teaspoon of turmeric powder with a cup of warm milk (dairy or plant-based), a pinch of black pepper, and a sweetener like honey or maple syrup.
2. **Smoothies:** Add 1/2 teaspoon of turmeric powder to your favorite smoothie. Combine with fruits like mango, pineapple, and banana for a tropical twist.

3. **Teas:** Brew turmeric tea by boiling 1 teaspoon of fresh grated turmeric or turmeric powder with water. Add lemon and honey for flavor.

4. **Cooking:** Use turmeric in soups, stews, curries, and rice dishes. It pairs well with spices like cumin, coriander, and ginger.

5. **Salad Dressings:** Mix turmeric powder into salad dressings for a vibrant color and health boost.

Topical Use

- **Turmeric Paste:** Create a paste with turmeric powder and water or coconut oil. Apply it to minor cuts, scrapes, or insect bites to take advantage of its antibacterial properties.

- **Face Masks:** Combine turmeric with yogurt or honey to make a face mask that can help reduce acne and improve skin tone.

Turmeric-Based Remedies and Recipes

Remedies

1. Cold and Flu Remedy: Combine turmeric with ginger, honey, and lemon juice in hot water to soothe symptoms and boost immunity.
2. Digestive Aid: A warm cup of turmeric tea before meals can help stimulate digestion and relieve bloating.
3. Joint Pain Relief: A paste made from turmeric and coconut oil applied to sore joints can reduce inflammation and pain.

Recipes

Turmeric Rice

- Ingredients: 1 cup basmati rice, 1 teaspoon turmeric powder, 2 cups water, salt to taste.
- Instructions: Rinse the rice and cook with water, turmeric, and salt until the rice is tender and fluffy.

Turmeric Hummus

- Ingredients: 1 can chickpeas, 1 teaspoon turmeric powder, 2 tablespoons tahini, 1 clove garlic, juice of 1 lemon, salt to taste, olive oil.
- Instructions: Blend all ingredients until smooth. Adjust seasoning and consistency with water or olive oil.

Turmeric Smoothie Bowl

- Ingredients: 1 frozen banana, 1/2 cup mango chunks, 1 teaspoon turmeric powder, 1 cup coconut milk, toppings (granola, chia seeds, fresh fruits).
- Instructions: Blend banana, mango, turmeric, and coconut milk until smooth. Pour into a bowl and top with desired toppings.

Potential Interactions and Contraindications of Turmeric

While turmeric is generally safe for most people, it can interact with certain medications and conditions:

Interactions

1. Blood Thinners: Turmeric can enhance the effects of blood-thinning medications (e.g., warfarin), increasing the risk of bleeding.
2. Diabetes Medications: It may lower blood sugar levels, which can interfere with diabetes management.
3. Stomach Acid Reducers: Turmeric might increase stomach acid production, counteracting the effects of medications that reduce stomach acid.

Contraindications

1. Gallbladder Problems: Turmeric can worsen gallbladder issues due to its effect on bile production.
2. Pregnancy and Breastfeeding: High doses of turmeric supplements are not recommended as they may stimulate the uterus or affect hormone levels.
3. Allergies: Some individuals may be allergic to turmeric or develop skin irritation from topical use.

Recommended Precautions

- **Consult a Healthcare Provider:** Especially if you are on medication or have underlying health conditions.
- **Moderation is Key:** While turmeric is beneficial, excessive consumption can lead to gastrointestinal issues and other side effects.
- **Quality Matters:** Use high-quality turmeric products to ensure purity and effectiveness.

By understanding the benefits, uses, and potential risks of turmeric, you can safely incorporate this powerful spice into your daily life and enjoy its numerous health benefits.

Chapter 10

Other Herbal Antibiotics

In addition to turmeric, many other herbs possess powerful antibiotic properties that have been utilized in traditional medicine for centuries. This chapter explores the unique properties and uses of some of these remarkable herbs, including Aloe vera, Calendula, Sage, Neem, and more.

Aloe Vera
Unique Properties

Aloe vera (Aloe barbadensis) is a succulent plant known for its soothing and healing properties. The gel found inside its leaves contains compounds such as polysaccharides, glycoproteins, and anthraquinones, which have antimicrobial and anti-inflammatory effects.

Uses

- Skin Infections and Wounds: Aloe vera gel is widely used to treat burns, cuts, and other skin infections due to its ability to accelerate wound healing and reduce inflammation.

- Digestive Health: Consuming Aloe vera juice can help alleviate gastrointestinal issues such as ulcers, irritable bowel syndrome (IBS), and constipation.
- Oral Health: Aloe vera mouthwash can reduce plaque and soothe gum inflammation.

Calendula
Unique Properties

Calendula (Calendula officinalis), also known as pot marigold, is renowned for its bright orange flowers and potent medicinal properties. It contains triterpenoids, flavonoids, and essential oils that provide anti-inflammatory, antiviral, and antibacterial benefits.

Uses

- Topical Applications: Calendula cream or ointment is effective in treating minor wounds, burns, rashes, and eczema.

- Oral Rinses: A calendula-infused rinse can help treat oral infections and soothe sore throats.
- Digestive Aid: Calendula tea can help alleviate stomach ulcers, indigestion, and menstrual cramps.

Sage
Unique Properties

Sage (Salvia officinalis) is a herb with a long history of medicinal use. Its antimicrobial properties are primarily due to its high content of essential oils, such as thujone, camphor, and cineole.

Uses

- Respiratory Health: Sage tea or inhalation of sage steam can relieve symptoms of respiratory infections, such as sore throats, coughs, and sinusitis.
- Skin Conditions: Sage-infused oil can be applied to treat acne, eczema, and fungal infections.
- Oral Health: Sage mouthwash is effective in reducing gum

inflammation, gingivitis, and bad breath.

Neem
Unique Properties

Neem (Azadirachta indica) is a tree native to India known for its powerful medicinal properties. Neem contains compounds such as azadirachtin, nimbin, and quercetin, which have strong antibacterial, antifungal, and antiviral effects.

Uses

- Skin Treatments: Neem oil is widely used to treat acne, eczema, psoriasis, and other skin infections due to its antibacterial and anti-inflammatory properties.
- Oral Hygiene: Neem-based toothpaste and mouthwash can help prevent dental plaque, cavities, and gum diseases.
- Internal Cleansing: Consuming neem supplements or tea can help detoxify the body, support liver function, and boost immunity.

Echinacea
Unique Properties

Echinacea (Echinacea purpurea) is a flowering plant often used to boost the immune system. It contains alkamides, glycoproteins, and polysaccharides, which contribute to its antimicrobial and immunostimulant effects.

Uses

- Cold and Flu Prevention: Echinacea supplements or tea can help reduce the duration and severity of colds and flu by enhancing immune response.
- Wound Healing: Topical application of Echinacea ointment can accelerate the healing of cuts, burns, and insect bites.
- Respiratory Health: Echinacea can be used to alleviate symptoms of respiratory infections such as bronchitis and sinusitis.

Garlic
Unique Properties

Garlic (Allium sativum) is a powerful natural antibiotic known for its broad-spectrum antimicrobial properties. The compound allicin, released when garlic is crushed or chopped, is responsible for its potent antibacterial and antifungal effects.

Uses

- Infection Prevention: Consuming raw garlic or garlic supplements can help prevent and treat various infections, including colds and urinary tract infections (UTIs).
- Heart Health: Garlic can lower blood pressure, reduce cholesterol levels, and improve overall cardiovascular health.
- Digestive Health: Garlic supports gut health by promoting the growth of beneficial bacteria and inhibiting harmful pathogens.

Thyme
Unique Properties

Thyme (Thymus vulgaris) is an herb known for its antiseptic and antimicrobial properties. It contains thymol and carvacrol, which are effective against a wide range of bacteria and fungi.

Uses

- Respiratory Infections: Thyme tea or inhalation of thyme steam can help relieve symptoms of bronchitis, coughs, and colds.
- Skin Conditions: Thyme-infused oil can be applied to treat fungal infections, acne, and minor wounds.
- Oral Health: Thyme mouthwash can help prevent tooth decay, gum disease, and bad breath.

Oregano
Unique Properties

Oregano (Origanum vulgare) is an herb with strong antimicrobial properties, primarily due to its high content of carvacrol and thymol. These compounds make oregano a powerful natural antibiotic.

Uses

- Digestive Health: Oregano oil can help treat digestive issues such as bloating, indigestion, and bacterial overgrowth.
- Respiratory Health: Oregano tea or oil can relieve symptoms of respiratory infections, including colds, flu, and bronchitis.
- Skin Infections: Oregano oil can be applied topically to treat fungal infections, wounds, and insect bites.

Conclusion

Herbal antibiotics offer a natural and effective way to prevent and treat a wide range of infections. Each herb has unique properties and uses, making them versatile tools in promoting health and well-being. By incorporating these powerful herbs into your daily routine, you can enhance your body's natural defenses and support overall health. Always consult with a healthcare provider before starting any new herbal regimen, especially if you have existing health conditions or are taking other medications.

Chapter 11

Combining Herbal Antibiotics for Maximum Effectiveness

Combining herbal antibiotics for maximum effectiveness involves understanding the properties of different herbs and how they can complement each other. Here are some key points to consider when combining herbal antibiotics:

Synergistic Effects: Look for herbs that have complementary actions or properties. For example, combining an herb with antimicrobial properties like garlic with an immune-boosting herb like Echinacea can enhance overall effectiveness against infections.

Broad Spectrum: Choose herbs with a broad spectrum of antimicrobial activity to target a wide range of pathogens. Herbs like oregano, thyme, and neem have broad-spectrum antimicrobial properties and can be effective when used together.

Dosage and Ratios: Pay attention to the appropriate dosages and ratios of each herb when combining them. Some herbs may require specific proportions to achieve synergistic effects while avoiding potential side effects.

Form of Administration: Consider how the herbs will be administered and whether they can be effectively combined in that form. For example, herbs can be taken orally as teas, tinctures, or capsules, or applied topically as ointments or creams.

Safety and Interactions: Ensure that the combined herbs do not have adverse interactions and are safe for the individual. Some herbs may have contraindications or interactions with certain medications, so it's essential to consult with a healthcare professional before combining them.

Balance and Moderation: Avoid over-reliance on any single herb and aim for a balanced combination that addresses specific health concerns while supporting overall well-being. Moderation is key to prevent overuse and potential side effects.

Personalization: Consider individual factors such as health status, age, and specific health goals when combining herbal antibiotics. What works well for one person may not be suitable for another, so it's essential to personalize the combination based on individual needs.

By carefully selecting and combining herbal antibiotics based on these principles, you can create potent and effective remedies that harness the full potential of medicinal herbs for maximum effectiveness against infections and overall health support. Always consult with a healthcare professional before starting any new herbal treatment regimen, especially if you have underlying health conditions or are taking other medications.

Understanding the Concept of Synergistic Effects

What Are Synergistic Effects?

Synergistic effects occur when two or more substances work together to produce a combined effect that is greater than the sum of their individual effects. In the context of herbal antibiotics, this means that certain herbs, when used together, can enhance each other's antibacterial, antiviral, and antifungal properties, resulting in more potent and effective remedies.

Benefits of Synergy in Herbal Medicine

1. Enhanced Efficacy: Combining herbs can boost their antimicrobial activity, making the treatment more effective against infections.
2. Broader Spectrum of Action: Using multiple herbs can target a wider range of pathogens, addressing various bacterial, viral, and fungal infections simultaneously.
3. Reduced Resistance: Pathogens are less likely to develop resistance to a combination of herbs compared to a single antimicrobial agent.
4. Balanced Effects: Synergistic combinations can mitigate potential side effects of individual herbs, creating a more balanced and tolerable treatment.

Guidelines for Combining Herbal Antibiotics

Principles to Follow

1. Complementary Actions: Choose herbs with complementary properties to enhance overall effectiveness. For example, combining an anti-inflammatory herb with an antimicrobial one can help reduce symptoms while fighting the infection.

2. Dosage and Ratios: Pay attention to the appropriate dosages and ratios of each herb to ensure safety and efficacy. Some herbs may require specific proportions to work synergistically.

3. Form of Administration: Consider how the herbs will be administered (e.g., tea, tincture, ointment) and whether they can be effectively combined in that form.

4. Safety and Interactions: Ensure that the combined herbs do not have adverse interactions and are safe for the individual, especially if they have

underlying health conditions or are taking other medications.

Common Combinations

1. Garlic and Echinacea: Garlic's potent antimicrobial properties combined with Echinacea's immune-boosting effects make this duo effective against colds and respiratory infections.
2. Turmeric and Ginger: Both have strong anti-inflammatory and antimicrobial properties, and together they can effectively treat digestive and respiratory infections.
3. Oregano and Thyme: Rich in thymol and carvacrol, this combination is powerful against bacterial and fungal infections.

Recipes and Remedies Using Multiple Herbal Antibiotics

Cold and Flu Tonic

Ingredients

- 1 cup water
- 1 teaspoon grated fresh ginger
- 1 teaspoon grated fresh turmeric

- 1 clove garlic, minced
- 1 teaspoon dried Echinacea
- 1 tablespoon honey
- Juice of 1 lemon

Instructions

1. Bring the water to a boil in a saucepan.
2. Add the ginger, turmeric, garlic, and Echinacea.
3. Reduce the heat and simmer for 10 minutes.
4. Strain the mixture into a cup.
5. Stir in the honey and lemon juice.
6. Drink while warm to help alleviate cold and flu symptoms.

Antimicrobial Skin Ointment

Ingredients

- 1/4 cup coconut oil
- 1 tablespoon beeswax
- 1 teaspoon neem oil
- 1 teaspoon calendula oil
- 5 drops tea tree oil
- 5 drops lavender essential oil

Instructions

1. In a double boiler, melt the coconut oil and beeswax together.
2. Remove from heat and stir in the neem oil, calendula oil, tea tree oil, and lavender essential oil.
3. Pour the mixture into a small jar and let it cool and solidify.
4. Apply the ointment to minor cuts, scrapes, and skin infections.

Digestive Health Tea

Ingredients

- 1 teaspoon dried peppermint leaves
- 1 teaspoon dried sage leaves
- 1 teaspoon dried chamomile flowers
- 1/2 teaspoon dried oregano
- 2 cups water
- Honey to taste (optional)

Instructions

1. Bring the water to a boil.
2. Add the peppermint, sage, chamomile, and oregano.
3. Remove from heat and let steep for 10 minutes.
4. Strain the tea into a cup.

5. Add honey if desired for sweetness.
6. Drink to help soothe digestive issues and support gut health.

Respiratory Relief Steam
Ingredients
- 1 teaspoon dried thyme
- 1 teaspoon dried rosemary
- 1 teaspoon dried eucalyptus leaves
- 4 cups boiling water

Instructions

1. Place the dried thyme, rosemary, and eucalyptus leaves in a large bowl.
2. Pour the boiling water over the herbs.
3. Lean over the bowl, covering your head with a towel to trap the steam.
4. Breathe deeply for 10-15 minutes to help relieve respiratory congestion and infections.

Immune-Boosting Elixir
Ingredients
- 1/2 cup apple cider vinegar
- 1/4 cup honey
- 1 tablespoon grated fresh horseradish
- 1 tablespoon grated fresh ginger

- 1 clove garlic, minced
- 1 teaspoon turmeric powder
- 1 teaspoon cayenne pepper

Instructions

1. Combine all ingredients in a jar and shake well.
2. Let the mixture sit for a week, shaking daily.
3. Strain the elixir into a clean jar.
4. Take 1-2 tablespoons daily to boost immune function and protect against infections.

Conclusion

Combining herbal antibiotics can significantly enhance their effectiveness, offering a powerful and natural approach to preventing and treating infections. By understanding the principles of synergy and following guidelines for safe and effective combinations, you can create potent remedies that harness the full potential of medicinal herbs. These recipes and remedies provide practical ways to incorporate multiple herbs into your health regimen, promoting overall wellness and resilience against pathogens. Always consult with a healthcare provider before starting new herbal treatments, especially if you have existing health conditions or are taking other medications.

Chapter 12

Safety and Precautions

Possible Side Effects and Contraindications of Herbal Antibiotics

While herbal antibiotics offer numerous health benefits, they are not without potential side effects and contraindications. Understanding these risks is crucial for safe and effective use.

Common Side Effects

1. Gastrointestinal Issues: Some herbs, such as garlic and oregano, can cause stomach upset, nausea, or diarrhea, especially when consumed in large amounts.
2. Allergic Reactions: Certain herbs may trigger allergic reactions in sensitive individuals. Symptoms can range from mild skin rashes to severe anaphylaxis.
3. Skin Irritation: Topical application of herbal extracts, like tea tree oil or

neem oil, can cause irritation or dermatitis in some people.
4. Photosensitivity: Herbs such as St. John's wort can increase sensitivity to sunlight, leading to a higher risk of sunburn.

Contraindications

1. Pregnancy and Breastfeeding: Some herbs, including turmeric and sage, can affect hormonal balance and uterine contractions, posing risks during pregnancy and breastfeeding.
2. Autoimmune Disorders: Herbs like Echinacea can stimulate the immune system, potentially exacerbating autoimmune conditions such as lupus or rheumatoid arthritis.
3. Blood Disorders: Garlic and ginger have blood-thinning properties, which can be problematic for individuals with bleeding disorders or those taking anticoagulant medications.
4. Chronic Conditions: Certain herbs may interact negatively with medications for chronic conditions such as diabetes, hypertension, or

heart disease. For example, ginseng can affect blood sugar levels and blood pressure.

Dosage Recommendations and Precautions

Proper dosage is critical to maximize the benefits of herbal antibiotics while minimizing the risk of side effects.

General Dosage Guidelines
1. Start Low and Go Slow: Begin with a low dose to assess tolerance, gradually increasing to the recommended amount.
2. Follow Standard Dosages: Adhere to dosage instructions provided on product labels or by healthcare professionals.
3. Herbal Teas: Typically, 1-2 teaspoons of dried herb per cup of water, consumed up to three times daily.
4. Tinctures: Commonly, 1-2 ml (about 30-60 drops) taken 2-3 times daily.
5. Capsules and Tablets: Follow the manufacturer's recommended dosage,

usually 1-2 capsules/tablets 1-3 times per day.

Specific Herb Precautions

1. Turmeric: High doses can cause stomach upset and, in rare cases, liver issues. Recommended daily intake is 500-2000 mg of turmeric extract.
2. Garlic: Excessive consumption may lead to gastrointestinal discomfort and bleeding risks. Limit intake to 1-2 cloves per day or follow supplement guidelines.
3. Echinacea: Prolonged use (over 8 weeks) may lead to immune system overactivation. Use intermittently, especially for cold and flu prevention.
4. Oregano Oil: Highly concentrated; use 1-4 drops diluted in water or carrier oil, up to three times daily. Avoid prolonged use due to potential liver strain.

Consulting with a Healthcare Professional

Importance of Professional Guidance

1. Accurate Diagnosis: A healthcare professional can provide a proper diagnosis and determine if herbal antibiotics are appropriate for your condition.
2. Personalized Advice: Tailored recommendations based on individual health status, medications, and potential herb-drug interactions.
3. Monitoring: Regular check-ups to monitor effectiveness and adjust dosages as needed.

When to Seek Advice

- Pre-existing Conditions: If you have chronic health issues or are taking prescription medications.
- Pregnancy and Breastfeeding: To ensure the safety of both mother and child.

- Severe Symptoms: If you experience severe side effects or allergic reactions.
- Long-term Use: For guidance on the safe duration of herbal antibiotic use.

Guidelines for Self-Management

Best Practices for Safe Use

1. Educate Yourself: Learn about the herbs you plan to use, including their benefits, side effects, and proper dosages.
2. Quality Products: Choose high-quality, reputable brands to ensure purity and potency.
3. Track Your Health: Keep a journal of your herbal antibiotic use, noting any changes in symptoms or side effects.
4. Moderation: Avoid excessive use; adhere to recommended dosages and durations.

Recognizing When to Seek Medical Attention

1. Persistent Symptoms: If symptoms do not improve or worsen after a few days of self-treatment.
2. Severe Reactions: Sudden onset of severe symptoms, such as difficulty breathing, swelling, or extreme dizziness.
3. Unusual Side Effects: Experiencing unexpected side effects not typically associated with the herb.

Tips for Safe Storage and Handling

- Proper Storage: Store herbs in a cool, dry place away from direct sunlight to maintain their potency.
- Shelf Life: Be aware of the shelf life of herbs and herbal products, discarding any that are expired or show signs of spoilage.
- Handling: Wash hands before and after handling herbs to prevent contamination and ensure safe topical application.

Conclusion

Herbal antibiotics can be a valuable addition to your health regimen, offering natural and effective alternatives to conventional antibiotics. However, safety and precaution are paramount to prevent adverse effects and ensure optimal outcomes. By understanding possible side effects, adhering to dosage recommendations, consulting with healthcare professionals, and following guidelines for self-management, you can safely harness the healing power of herbal antibiotics. Always prioritize your health and well-being by making informed decisions and seeking professional advice when necessary.

Conclusion

Recap of the Benefits of Herbal Antibiotics

Throughout this book, we have explored the remarkable world of herbal antibiotics, understanding their profound benefits and diverse applications. Here are the key takeaways:

Natural and Effective

Herbal antibiotics offer a natural alternative to synthetic antibiotics, leveraging the medicinal properties of plants to combat a wide range of infections. They are effective against bacteria, viruses, and fungi, providing a holistic approach to health and wellness.

Fewer Side Effects

Compared to conventional antibiotics, herbal antibiotics typically have fewer and less severe side effects. They are less likely to disrupt the natural balance of the body, preserving beneficial bacteria and reducing the risk of antibiotic resistance.

Multi-functional Benefits

Many herbal antibiotics not only fight infections but also offer additional health benefits, such as anti-inflammatory, antioxidant, and immune-boosting properties. This makes them versatile tools for promoting overall health and preventing illness.

Sustainable and Accessible

Herbal antibiotics are often more sustainable and accessible than their pharmaceutical counterparts. Many herbs can be grown at home or purchased from local markets, empowering individuals to take charge of their health in a cost-effective and environmentally friendly way.

Encouragement to Explore the World of Herbal Remedies

Embarking on a journey into the world of herbal remedies can be incredibly rewarding. Here are some steps and encouragements to guide you:

Start Small

Begin with a few well-researched herbs that are known for their safety and effectiveness. As you gain confidence and knowledge, gradually expand your herbal repertoire.

Educate Yourself

Knowledge is power. Read books, attend workshops, and consult reputable sources to deepen your understanding of herbal medicine. This book serves as a foundation, but the field of herbalism is vast and continually evolving.

Experiment and Personalize

Each individual responds differently to herbal treatments. Experiment with different herbs and combinations to find what works best for your unique needs. Keep a journal to track your experiences and outcomes.

Connect with the Community

Join local or online herbalist communities to share experiences, ask questions, and learn from others. The support and wisdom of a community can enhance your journey and provide valuable insights.

Final Thoughts on Harnessing the Potency of Herbal Antibiotics

Harnessing the potency of herbal antibiotics is both an art and a science. It requires a balance of knowledge, intuition, and respect for the natural world. Here are some final thoughts to inspire and guide you:

Respect Nature's Wisdom

Herbal antibiotics are gifts from nature, offering powerful healing properties derived from plants. Approach them with respect and gratitude, acknowledging the centuries of traditional knowledge that underpin their use.

Integrate Holistically

Herbal antibiotics are most effective when integrated into a holistic approach to health. Combine them with a balanced diet, regular exercise, sufficient rest, and stress management to support your body's natural healing processes.

Seek Balance

Moderation and balance are key in herbal medicine. Avoid over-reliance on any single herb or remedy. Instead, aim for a diverse and balanced approach that supports overall health and prevents overuse.

Stay Informed

Stay informed about the latest research and developments in herbal medicine. The field is dynamic, with ongoing studies uncovering new benefits and applications for herbal antibiotics.

Empower Yourself

Taking charge of your health through the use of herbal antibiotics is empowering. It fosters a deeper connection with your body and the natural world, promoting a proactive and preventive approach to well-being.

Conclusion

Herbal antibiotics offer a natural, effective, and sustainable way to enhance health and combat infections. By understanding their benefits, exploring the vast world of herbal remedies, and harnessing their potency with respect and knowledge, you can unlock the full potential of these remarkable natural medicines. Embrace the journey, stay curious, and let the wisdom of herbs guide you towards a healthier, more balanced life.

Appendix: Quick Reference Guide

Summary of Herbal Antibiotics and Their Uses

Aloe Vera
- **Uses:** Skin infections, wounds, burns, digestive health, oral health
- **Properties:** Antimicrobial, anti-inflammatory

Calendula
- **Uses:** Wounds, burns, rashes, eczema, oral rinses, digestive aid
- **Properties:** Antibacterial, antiviral, anti-inflammatory

Sage
- Uses: Respiratory infections, skin conditions, oral health
- Properties: Antimicrobial, antiseptic, anti-inflammatory

Neem
- Uses: Skin treatments, oral hygiene, internal cleansing

- Properties: Antibacterial, antifungal, antiviral

Echinacea
- Uses: Cold and flu prevention, wound healing, respiratory health
- Properties: Immunostimulant, antimicrobial

Garlic
- Uses: Infection prevention, heart health, digestive health
- Properties: Antibacterial, antifungal, antiviral

Thyme
- Uses: Respiratory infections, skin conditions, oral health
- Properties: Antiseptic, antimicrobial

Oregano
- Uses: Digestive health, respiratory health, skin infections
- Properties: Antibacterial, antifungal

Dosage Guidelines for Each Herb

Aloe Vera

- Topical: Apply aloe vera gel directly to the affected area 2-3 times daily.
- Oral: Drink 1/4 cup of aloe vera juice 1-2 times daily.

Calendula

- Topical: Apply calendula ointment or cream to the affected area 2-3 times daily.
- Oral: Drink calendula tea (1-2 teaspoons of dried flowers per cup of water) up to 3 times daily.

Sage

- Topical: Apply sage-infused oil to the skin 2-3 times daily.
- Oral: Use sage tea (1 teaspoon of dried leaves per cup of water) up to 3 times daily, or use as a mouthwash.

Neem

- Topical: Apply neem oil to the affected area once or twice daily.

- Oral: Take neem supplements as directed, usually 1-2 capsules per day, or drink neem tea (1 teaspoon of dried leaves per cup of water) once daily.

Echinacea

- Oral: Take Echinacea tincture (1-2 ml) or capsules (300-500 mg) 2-3 times daily for up to 8 weeks.

Garlic

- Oral: Eat 1-2 cloves of raw garlic per day, or take garlic supplements (600-1200 mg) divided into multiple doses daily.

Thyme

- Topical: Apply thyme-infused oil to the affected area 2-3 times daily.
- Oral: Drink thyme tea (1 teaspoon of dried leaves per cup of water) up to 3 times daily.

Oregano

- Oral: Take oregano oil (1-4 drops diluted in water or juice) up to 3 times daily.

- Topical: Dilute oregano oil in a carrier oil (1:10 ratio) and apply to the skin 2-3 times daily.

Tips for Incorporating Herbal Antibiotics into Your Routine

Start with Familiar Herbs

- Begin with herbs you are already familiar with, such as garlic or aloe vera, and gradually introduce new ones into your routine.

Consistent Usage

- For preventive health, incorporate herbal antibiotics into your daily routine consistently. For acute infections, follow the recommended dosages closely until symptoms improve.

Diversify Your Herbs

- Use a variety of herbs to avoid over-reliance on a single type. This can prevent the body from developing resistance and ensure a broad spectrum of benefits.

Form Integration

- Choose the form that best fits your lifestyle and preference. For example, teas and tinctures are convenient for oral intake, while oils and creams are suitable for topical application.

Monitor Your Health

- Keep track of any changes in your health, noting improvements or any adverse reactions. Adjust your usage based on your observations and consult with a healthcare professional if necessary.

Combine with a Healthy Lifestyle

- Enhance the effectiveness of herbal antibiotics by maintaining a healthy diet, staying hydrated, getting regular exercise, and managing stress.

Educate and Consult

- Continuously educate yourself about the herbs you use and consult with a healthcare professional, especially if you have underlying health conditions or are taking other medications.

By following these guidelines and recommendations, you can safely and effectively integrate herbal antibiotics into your daily routine, harnessing their natural potency to support your overall health and well-being.

Glossary

Definitions of Key Terms Used in the Book

Adaptogen

A natural substance considered to help the body adapt to stress and exert a normalizing effect upon bodily processes. Examples include ashwagandha and ginseng.

Antibacterial

A substance that kills bacteria or inhibits their growth. Herbal antibiotics like garlic and thyme have strong antibacterial properties.

Antifungal

A substance that kills fungi or inhibits their growth. Neem and oregano are known for their antifungal capabilities.

Antimicrobial

A broad term that refers to any substance that kills or inhibits the growth of microorganisms, including bacteria, viruses, and fungi.

Antioxidant

A substance that inhibits oxidation or reactions promoted by oxygen, peroxides, or free radicals. Turmeric and green tea are rich in antioxidants.

Antiseptic

A substance that prevents or arrests the growth of microorganisms, typically applied to living tissues. Sage and thyme are often used as antiseptics.

Antiviral

A substance that inhibits the growth of viruses. Echinacea and elderberry have antiviral properties.

Carminative

A substance that helps expel gas from the intestines, thereby relieving bloating and discomfort. Ginger and peppermint are common carminatives.

Contraindication

A specific situation or condition where a particular treatment or medication should not be used because it may be harmful. For example, using certain herbs during pregnancy might be contraindicated.

Decoction

A method of extraction by boiling plant material (roots, bark, and other dense parts) to dissolve the chemicals of the material. This is commonly used for hard and woody substances.

Essential Oil

A concentrated hydrophobic liquid containing volatile chemical compounds from plants. Essential oils of oregano and tea tree are used for their antimicrobial properties.

Herbal Antibiotic

A plant-derived substance used to treat or prevent bacterial infections. Examples include garlic, turmeric, and Echinacea.

Immune Stimulant

A substance that stimulates the immune system to increase its activity against pathogens. Echinacea and astragalus are known immune stimulants.

Infusion

A method of extracting chemical compounds from plants by steeping them in hot water, similar to making tea. This method is often used for leaves, flowers, and other soft plant parts.

Maceration

The process of soaking plant material in a liquid (usually alcohol, water, or oil) to extract its medicinal compounds over a longer period without heat.

Phytochemical

A bioactive chemical compound that occurs naturally in plants. These compounds often have beneficial health effects, such as the curcuminoids in turmeric.

Poultice

A soft, moist mass of plant material applied to the body to relieve soreness and inflammation and improve healing.

Synergy

The interaction of two or more substances to produce a combined effect greater than the sum of their separate effects. In herbal medicine, combining herbs can enhance their overall therapeutic effect.

Tincture

An extract of a plant made by soaking herbs in a solvent, usually alcohol or glycerin. Tinctures are potent and have a long shelf life.

Volatile Oil

An oil that evaporates readily at normal temperatures and is usually extracted by distillation. Essential oils are types of volatile oils.

Adaptogen

Herbs or substances that help the body adapt to stress and promote balance and homeostasis. Examples include ashwagandha and Rhodiola.

Anti-inflammatory

A substance that reduces inflammation in the body. Turmeric and ginger are well-known anti-inflammatory herbs.

Decoction

A method of extraction by boiling plant material (roots, bark, and other dense parts) to dissolve the chemicals of the material. This is commonly used for hard and woody substances.

Efficacy

The ability to produce a desired or intended result. In the context of herbal antibiotics, it refers to how effective the herb is at treating infections.

Extraction

The process of obtaining active ingredients from plants. Methods include infusion, decoction, maceration, and tincturing.

Immunomodulator

A substance that helps regulate or normalize the immune system. Some herbs, like Echinacea, can act as immunomodulators.

Mucilage

A thick, gluey substance produced by nearly all plants and some microorganisms. It has soothing and protective properties, often used in herbal medicine to treat irritated tissues.

Phytotherapy

The use of plant-derived medications in the treatment and prevention of diseases. This term is often used interchangeably with herbal medicine.

Standardized Extract

An herbal extract that has a consistent concentration of specific active ingredients. This ensures uniformity and reliability in the product's effects.

Terpene

A large and diverse class of organic compounds produced by a variety of plants, especially conifers. Terpenes often have strong odors and can have therapeutic properties.

Therapeutic Dose

The amount of a substance required to achieve the desired therapeutic effect. Determining the therapeutic dose is essential for the safe and effective use of herbal antibiotics.

Tonic

A medicinal substance taken to give a feeling of vigor or well-being. Tonics are often used to strengthen and invigorate organs or bodily systems.

Vulnerary

A substance that promotes the healing of wounds or cuts. Calendula and aloe vera are examples of herbs with vulnerary properties.